The Complete Dash Diet Cooking Plan

A Collection of Delicious Dishes Easy to Prepare!

Natalie Puckett

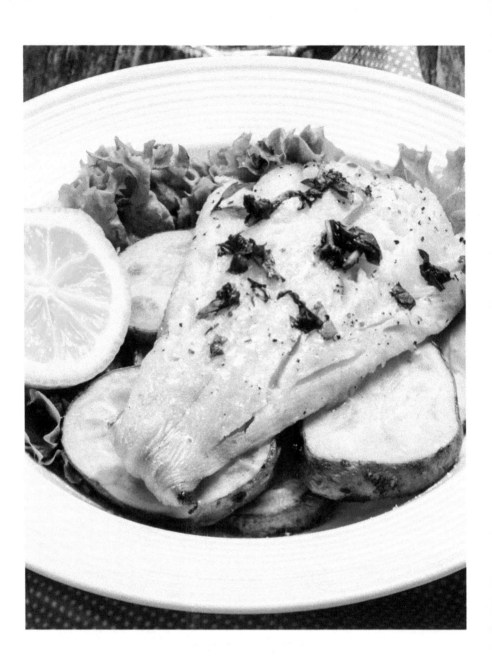

Table of Contents

Grilled Cod Fillets with Lemon Dill Butter

SmartPoints value: Green plan - 3SP, Blue plan - 2SP, Purple plan - 2SP

Total Time: 25 min, Prep time: 15 min, Cooking time: 10 min, Serves: 4

Nutritional value: Calories - 318.7g, Carbs - 6.7g, Fat - 13.0g, Protein - 41.7g

Ingredients

Olive oil -2 tsp

Uncooked Atlantic cod - 24 oz, or another firm white fish like

tilapia (four 6-oz fillets)

Table salt - ½ tsp

Lemon(s) (sliced 1/4-in thick) - 2 medium (you'll need 12 slices total)

Dill - 2 tsp, chopped

Dill - 4 sprig(s)

Light butter - 4 tsp (at room temp.)

Lemon zest - 1 tsp

Instructions

1.   Get your grill ready by preheating to medium-high heat. Continue the heating for at least 10 minutes after it reaches the desired temperature, then scrape the grate clean with a steel brush and coat it lightly with oil.

2.   While the grill heats up, pat the fish dry and sprinkle salt on it.

3.   Place three lemon slices on the grill carefully, overlapping slightly, and top it with a dill sprig and fish fillet.

4.   Repeat the same with the remaining lemon, dill, and fish. Cover the grill and cook without turning for 8-10 minutes until the fish is opaque all the way through and yields easily to a thin-bladed knife.

5.   While the cooking is on-going, mix the butter, chopped dill, and zest in a small shallow bowl.

6.   Transfer each lemon-dill-fish portion to a plate using two thin-bladed spatulas and top them with 1 1/2 tsp of lemon-dill butter and serve (serving the lemon slices is optional).

Spicy Baked Shrimp

Serving: 4

Prep Time: 10 minutes

Cook Time: 25 minutes + 2-4 hours

Ingredients:

½ ounce large shrimp, peeled and deveined Cooking spray as needed

1 teaspoon low sodium coconut amines

1 teaspoon parsley

½ teaspoon olive oil

½ tablespoon honey

1 tablespoon lemon juice

How To:

1.   Pre-heat your oven to 450 degrees F.

2.   Take a baking dish and grease it well.

3.   Mix altogether the ingredients and toss.

4. Transfer to oven and bake for 8 minutes until shrimp turns pink.

5. Serve and enjoy!

Nutrition (Per Serving)

Calories: 321

Fat: 9g

Carbohydrates: 44g

Protein: 22g

Shrimp and Cilantro Meal

Serving: 4

Prep Time: 10 minutes

Cook Time: 5 minutes

Ingredients:

¾ pounds shrimp, deveined and peeled

tablespoons fresh lime juice

¼ teaspoon cloves, minced

½ teaspoon ground cumin

1 tablespoon olive oil

1 ¼ cups fresh cilantro, chopped

1 teaspoon lime zest

½ teaspoon sunflower seeds

¼ teaspoon pepper

Direction

1.   Take an outsized sized bowl and add shrimp, cumin, garlic, juice, ginger and toss well.

2.   Take an outsized sized non-stick skillet and add oil, allow the oil to heat up over medium-high heat.

3.   Add shrimp mixture and sauté for 4 minutes.

4.   Remove the warmth and add cilantro, lime zest, sunflower seeds, and pepper.

5.   Mix well and serve hot!

Nutrition (Per Serving)

Calories: 177

Fat: 6g

Carbohydrates: 2g

Protein: 27g

The Original Dijon Fish

Serving: 2

Prep Time: 3 minutes

Cook Time: 12 minutes

Ingredients:

1 perch, flounder or sole fish florets

1 tablespoon Dijon mustard

1 ½ teaspoons lemon juice

teaspoon low sodium Worcestershire sauce, low sodium tablespoons Italian seasoned bread crumbs 1 almond butter flavored cooking spray

How To:

1.   Preheat your oven to 450 degrees F.

2.   Take an 11 x 7-inch baking dish and arrange your fillets carefully.

3.   Take a little sized bowl and add juice, Worcester sauce, mustard and blend it well.

4.   Pour the combination over your fillet.

5. Sprinkle an honest amount of breadcrumbs.

6. Bake for 12 minutes until fish flakes off easily.

7. Cut the fillet in half portions and enjoy!

Nutrition (Per Serving)

Calories: 125

Fat: 2g

Carbohydrates: 6g

Protein: 21g

Lemony Garlic Shrimp

Serving: 4

Prep Time: 5-10 minutes

Cook Time: 10-15 minutes

Ingredients:

1 ¼ pounds shrimp, boiled or steamed

tablespoons garlic, minced

¼ cup lemon juice

tablespoons olive oil

¼ cup parsley

How To:

1.   Take alittle skillet and place over medium heat, add garlic and oil and stir-cook for 1 minute.

2.   Add parsley, juice and season with sunflower seeds and pepper accordingly.

3.   Add shrimp during a large bowl and transfer the mixture from the skillet over the shrimp.

4.   Chill and serve.

5.   Enjoy!

Nutrition (Per Serving)

Calories: 130

Fat: 3g

Carbohydrates:2g

Protein:22g

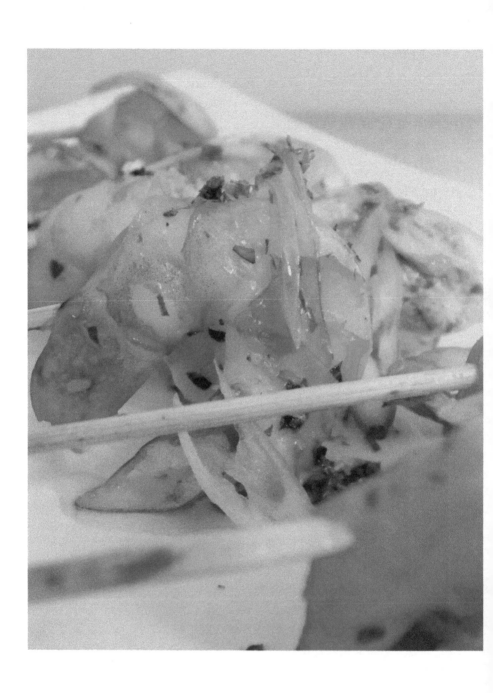

Chicken Tortilla Soup

SmartPoints value: Green plan - 4SP, Blue plan - 2SP, Purple plan - 2SP

Total Time: 45 min, Prep time: 15 min, Cooking time: 30 min, Serves: 6

Nutritional value:

Calories - 200, Carbs - 24g, Fat - 9g, Protein - 7g

Ingredients

Cilantro (chopped) - 1 cup(s)

Chili powder - 1 tsp

Chicken broth (reduced-sodium) - 6 cup(s)

Olive oil - 1 tsp

Uncooked onion(s) (chopped) - 1½ cup(s)

Kosher salt -1½ tsp

Minced Garlic - 4 tsp

Jalapeño pepper(s) - 1 medium (seeded and minced)

Tomatoes (canned, diced)- 15 oz, fire roasted-variety, drained

Uncooked chicken breast - 20 oz (boneless, skinless)

Lime juice (fresh) - ⅓ cup(s)

Mexican-style cheese (Shredded reduced) - 6 Tbsp

Tortilla chips (crushed) - 12 chip(s)

Instructions

1. Set a soup pot over medium heat and preheat.

2. Toss in the chopped onion and salt, then cook, often stirring, until the onion gets soft; 5-10 minutes.

3. Add garlic, chili powder, and jalapeno, then cook for one minute.

4. Put in your broth, tomatoes, lime juice, and chicken, then stir to combine.

5. Simmer and cook until the chicken breasts cook through; about 20 minutes.

6. Remove the chicken breasts from the soup and shred them with two forks, then return the shredded chicken to the pot with cilantro.

7. Serve your soup garnished with tortilla chips and cheese.

Chicken Piccata Stir-Fry

SmartPoints value: Green plan - 4SP, Blue plan - 2SP, Purple plan - 2SP

Total Time: 25 min, Prep time: 20 min, Cooking time: 5 min, Serves: 4

Nutritional value: Cal - 190.5, Carbs - 5.6g, Fat - 9.4g, Protein - 18.6g

This dish is a combination of the classic Italian chicken piccata and Asian stir-fry.

Ingredients

Black pepper (freshly ground) - ¼ tsp

Capers (rinsed)- 1 Tbsp

Chicken broth (fat-free) - ½ cup(s)

Cornstarch (divided) - 2 tsp

Dry sherry (divided)- 3 Tbsp

Table salt (divided) - ¾ tsp

Soy sauce (low sodium) - 1 Tbsp

Peanut oil (divided) - 4 tsp, or vegetable oil

Uncooked chicken breast (boneless, skinless) - 1 pound(s), cut into quarter-inch-thick slices

Uncooked shallot(s) - 1 medium, thinly sliced Minced Garlic - 1 Tbsp

String beans (uncooked) - 2 cup(s), cut into two-inch lengths Parsley (fresh, chopped) - 2 Tbsp

Lemon(s) - ½ medium, cut into four

Instructions

1.   Prepare a clean medium-sized bowl and mix chicken, 1 tsp of cornstarch,1 Tbsp of dry sherry,1/2 tsp salt, and pepper in it.

2.   Next, get a small bowl and combine broth, soy sauce, remaining 2 Tbsp of dry sherry, and 1 tsp of cornstarch.

3.   Preheat a fourteen-inch flat-bottomed wok or twelve-inch skillet over high heat to the point where a drop of water will evaporate within 1 to 2 seconds of contact, then swirl in one Tbsp oil.

4.   Add shallots and garlic, then stir-fry for 10 seconds. Push the shallot mixture to the sides of the wok and add the chicken, then spread in one layer in the wok.

5.   Cook the chicken undisturbed for 60 seconds, allowing the chicken to begin searing, then stir-fry another 60 seconds until chicken is no longer pink but not yet thoroughly cooked.

6.   Swirl the chicken in the remaining 1 tsp oil and toss in green beans and capers. Sprinkle on the remaining 1/4 tsp of salt and stir-fry for 30 seconds or until just combined.

7.   Swirl the chicken in the broth mixture and stir-fry for 1-2 minutes or until the chicken is cooked through, with the sauce slightly thickened.

8.   Sprinkle the parsley on it and serve with lemon wedges.

Ranch Meatballs

SmartPoints value: Green plan - 4SP, Blue plan - 4SP, Purple plan – 5SP

Total Time: 20mins, Prep time: 10 mins, Cooking time: 30mins, Serves: 4

Nutritional value: Calories - 195, Carbs - 6g, Fat - 6g, Protein - 26g

Meatball recipes are delicious protein recipes that are so satisfying and tasty. They can be a fun and easy meal. It becomes easier to prepare the perfect sized meatballs using a meatball shaper.

Ingredients

Ground beef (96/4) (extra lean) - 1 lb

Panko breadcrumbs - 1/3 cup(s)

Egg substitute (Liquid, like egg beaters) - 1/4 cup

Olive oil - 1 tsp

Onion powder - 1 tbsp

Garlic powder - 1 tbsp

Dill (dried) - 2 tsp

Parsley (dried) - 2 tsp

Basil (dried) - 2 tsp

Salt and pepper - Add to taste

Instructions

1.   Combine all the ingredients by hand in a large bowl and shape it into about 24 meatballs.

2.   Apply heat to the oil in a large non-stick skillet over medium-high heat.

3.   Place meatballs in the pan and cook for about 1-2 minutes on each side, until all sides get lightly browned.

4.   Reduce the heat to medium-low and pour in half a cup of water. Cover it and cook, occasionally stirring, until meatballs cook thoroughly; about 10-12 minutes.

Note: Meatballs are a perfect simple Weight Watchers dinner recipe for those who are watching Points but also savour the flavour

Beef Orzo with Feta

SmartPoints value: Green plan - 8SP, Blue plan - 8SP, Purple plan – 8SP

Total Time: 35mins, Prep time: 10mins, Cooking time: 25mins, Serves: 6

Nutritional value: Calories - 325, Carbs – 44g, Fat – 5.5g, Protein – 25g

Ingredients

Ground beef (extra-lean) - 1 lb

Whole wheat orzo - 10 oz

Onion (finely chopped) - 1 large

Garlic (minced) - 4 cloves

Cinnamon (ground) - 1 tsp

Oregano (dried) - 2 tsp

Can tomatoes (crushed) - One 26oz

Reduced-fat feta cheese (crumbled) - 1/3 cup

Salt & pepper - Add to taste

Instructions

1.   Prepare whole orzo wheat according to package directions. Drain it and set aside.

2.   While the wheat is cooking, spray a large skillet with nonfat cooking spray, and set it over medium-high heat. Toss in some beef and cook until it mostly cooks through.

3.   Put in onions, oregano, garlic, cinnamon, salt, and pepper. Sauté the dish until the onions are tender and the beef cooks all the way through.

4.   Pour the crushed tomatoes into the skillet with the beef mixture, and cook on medium heat. Continue to cook, while occasionally stirring, until the mixture thickens; about 15 minutes.

5.   Dish the beef sauce with orzo and place in serving bowls. Top each bowl with 1 tbsp of feta.

Gentle Blackberry Crumble

Serving: 4

Prep Time: 10 minutes

Cook Time: 45 minutes

Smart Points: 4

Ingredients:

½ cup coconut flour

½ cup banana, peeled and mashed

6 tablespoons water

3 cups fresh blackberries

½ cup arrowroot flour

1 ½ teaspoons baking soda

4 tablespoons almond butter, melted

1 tablespoon fresh lemon juice

How To:

1.   Pre-heat your oven to 300 degrees F

2.   Take a baking dish and grease it lightly.

3.   Take a bowl and mix all of the ingredients except the blackberries, mix well.

4.   Place blackberries in the bottom of your baking dish and top with flour.

5.   Bake for 40 minutes.

6.   Serve and enjoy!

Nutrition (Per Serving)

Calories: 12

Fat: 7g

Carbohydrates: 10g

Protein: 4g

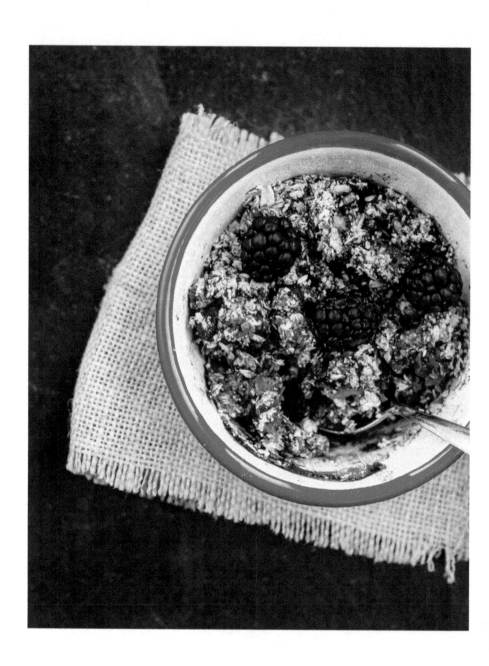

Mini Minty Happiness

Serving: 12

Prep Time: 45 minutes

Cooking Time: None Freeze Time: 2 hours

Ingredients:

2 teaspoons vanilla extract

1 ½ cups coconut oil

1 ¼ cups sunflower seed almond butter ½ cup dried parsley

1 teaspoon peppermint extract

A pinch of sunflower seeds

1 cup dark chocolate chips Stevia to taste

How To:

1.   Melt together coconut oil and dark chocolate chips over a double boiler.

2.   Take a food processor, add all the ingredients into it and pulse until smooth.

3.   Pour into round molds.

4.   Let it freeze.

Nutrition (Per Serving)

Total Carbs: 7g

Fiber: 1g

Protein: 3g

Fat: 25g

Astonishing Maple Pecan

Bacon Slices

Serving: 12

Prep Time: 10 minutes

Cooking Time: 25 minutes

Freeze Time: None

Ingredients:

tablespoon sugar-free maple syrup

12 bacon slices

Granulated Stevia to taste

15-20 drops Stevia For the coating:

4 tablespoons dark cocoa powder

¼ cup pecans, chopped

15-20 drops Stevia

How To:

1.   Take a baking tray and lay the bacon slices on it.

2.   Rub with maple syrup and Stevia, flip the slices and do the same with the other side.

3.   Bake for 10-15 minutes at 227 degrees F.

4.   After they've baked, drain the bacon grease.

5.   To form a batter, mix the bacon grease, Stevia and cocoa powder.

6.   Dip the bacon slices into the batter and roll in the chopped pecans.

7.   Allow to air dry until the chocolate hardens.

Nutrition (Per Serving)

Total Carbs: 1g

Fiber: 0g

Protein: 10g

Fat: 11g

Generous Maple and Pecan Bites

Serving: 12

Prep Time: 10 minutes

Cooking Time: 25 minutes

Freeze Time: None

Ingredients:

1 cup almond meal

½ cup coconut oil

½ cup flaxseed meal

½ cup sugar-free chocolate chips

2 cups pecans, chopped

½ cup sugar-free maple syrup

20-25 drops Stevia

How To:

1.   Take a baking dish and spread the pecans.

2.   Bake at 350 degrees F until aromatic.

3.   This will usually take from 6 to 8 minutes.

4.   Meanwhile, sift together all the dry ingredients.

5.   Add the roasted pecans to the mix and mix them properly.

6.   Add the coconut oil and maple syrup.

7.   Stir to make a thick, sticky mixture.

8.   Take a bread pan lined with parchment paper, and pour the mixture into it.

9.   Bake for about 18 minutes.

10.   Slice and serve.

Nutrition (Per Serving)

Total Carbs: 6g

Fiber: 0g

Protein: 5g

Fat: 30g

Carrot Ball Delight

Serving: 4

Prep Time: 10 minutes

Cook Time: Nil

Ingredients:

6 Medjool dates pitted

1 carrot, finely grated

¼ cup raw walnuts

¼ cup unsweetened coconut, shredded

1 teaspoon nutmeg

1/8 teaspoon sunflower seeds

How To:

1.   Take a food processor and add dates, ¼ cup of grated carrots, sunflower seeds coconut, nutmeg.

2.   Mix well and puree the mixture.

3.   Add the walnuts and remaining ¼ cup of carrots.

4.   Pulse the mixture until you have a chunky texture.

5.   Form balls using your hand and roll them up in coconut.

6.   Top with carrots and chill.

7.   Enjoy!

Nutrition (Per Serving)

Calories: 326

Fat: 16g

Carbohydrates: 42g

Protein: 3g

Awesome Brownie Muffins

Serving: 5

Prep Time: 10 minutes

Cooking Time: 35 minutes

Ingredients:

1 cup golden flaxseed meal

¼ cup cocoa powder

1 tablespoon cinnamon

½ tablespoon baking powder

½ teaspoon sunflower seeds

1 whole large egg

2 tablespoons coconut oil

¼ cup sugar-free caramel syrup

½ cup pumpkin puree

1 teaspoon vanilla extract

1 teaspoon apple cider vinegar

¼ cup almonds, slivered

How To:

1.   Pre-heat your oven to 350 degrees F.

2.   Take a mixing bowl and add all of the listed ingredients and mix everything well.

3.   Take your desired number of muffin tins and line them with paper liners.

4.   Scoop the batter into the muffin tins, filling them to about 1/4 of the liner.

5.   Sprinkle a bit of almond on top.

6.   Place them in your oven and bake for 15 minutes.

7.   Serve warm.

Nutrition (Per Serving)

Total Carbs: 16

Fiber: 2g

Protein: 3g

Fat: 31g

Spice Friendly Muffins

Serving: 12

Prep Time: 5 minutes

Cooking Time: 45minute

Ingredients:

½ cup raw hemp hearts

½ cup flaxseeds

¼ cup chia seeds

2 tablespoons Psyllium husk powder

1 tablespoon cinnamon

Stevia taste

½ teaspoon baking powder

½ teaspoon sunflower seeds

1 cup of water

How To:

1.   Pre-heat your oven to 350 degrees F.
2.

2.   Line muffin tray with liners.

3.   Take a large sized mixing bowl and add peanut almond butter, pumpkin, sweetener, coconut almond milk, flaxseed and mix well.

4.   Keep stirring until the mixture has been thoroughly combined.

5.   Take another bowl and add baking powder, spices and coconut flour.

6.   Mix well.

7.   Add the dry ingredients into the wet bowl and stir until the coconut flour has mixed well.

8.   Allow it to sit for a while until the coconut flour has absorbed all of the moisture.

9.   Divide the mixture amongst your muffin tins and bake for 45 minutes.

10.   Enjoy!

Nutrition (Per Serving)

Total Carbs: 7g

Fiber: 3g

Protein: 6g

Fat: 15g

Spicy Apple Crisp

Nutritional Facts

servings per container	5
Prep Total	**10 min**
Serving Size	7
Amount per serving **Calories**	**0.2%**
	% Daily Value
Total Fat 8g	**22%**
Saturated Fat 1g	51%
Trans Fat 0g	2%
Cholesterol	**2%**
Sodium 20mg	**0.2%**
Total Carbohydrate 70g	**540%**
Dietary Fiber 3g	1%
Total Sugar 6g	1%
Protein 6g	24
Vitamin C 4mcg	170%
Calcium 160mg	12%
Iron 2mg	210%
Potassium 30mg	21%

Ingredients:

8 cooking apples

4 oz or 150 g flour

7 oz or 350 g brown sugar

5 oz or 175 g vegan butter

¼ tablespoon ground cinnamon

¼ tablespoon ground nutmeg

Zest of one lemon

1 tablespoon fresh lemon juice

Instructions:

Peel, quarter and core cooking apples.

Cut apple quarters into thin slices and place them in a bowl.

Blend nutmeg and cinnamon then sprinkle over apples.

Sprinkle with lemon rind.

Add lemon juice and toss to blend.

Arrange slices in a large baking dish.

Make a mixture of sugar, flour, and vegan butter in a mixing bowl then put over apples, smoothing it over.

Place the dish in the oven.

Bake at 370°F, 190°C or gas mark 5 for 60 minutes, until browned and apples are tender.

Apple Cake

Nutritional Facts

servings per container	8
Prep Total	**10 min**
Serving Size	2
Amount per serving **Calories**	**0%**
	% Daily Value
Total Fat 4g	**210%**
Saturated Fat 3g	32%
Trans Fat 2g	2%
Cholesterol	**8%**
Sodium 300mg	**0.2%**
Total Carbohydrate 20g	**50%**
Dietary Fiber 1g	1%
Total Sugar 1g	1%
Protein 3g	
Vitamin C 1mcg	18%
Calcium 20mg	1%
Iron 8mg	12%
Potassium 70mg	21%

Ingredients:

2 oz or 50 g flour

3 tablespoon baking powder

½ tablespoon of salt

2 tablespoon vegan shortening

¼ pint or 125 ml unsweetened soya milk 4 or 5 apples

4 oz or 110 g sugar

1 tablespoon cinnamon

Instructions:

Sift together flour, baking powder, and salt.

Add shortening and rub in very lightly.

Add milk slowly to make soft dough and mix.

Place on floured board and roll out ½ inch or 1 cm thick.

Put into shallow greased pan.

Wash, pare, core, \ and cut apples into sections; press them into a dough.

Sprinkle with sugar and dust with cinnamon.

Bake at 375°F, 190°C, or gas mark 5 for 30 minutes or until apples are tender and brown.

Serve with soya cream.

Apple Charlotte

Nutritional Facts

servings per container	5
Prep Total	**10 min**
Serving Size	4
Amount per serving **Calories**	**60%**
	% Daily Value
Total Fat 1g	**200%**
Saturated Fat 20g	3%
Trans Fat 14g	2%
Cholesterol	**2%**
Sodium 210mg	**2%**
Total Carbohydrate 7g	**210%**
Dietary Fiber 1g	9%
Total Sugar 21g	8%
Protein 4g	
Vitamin C 4mcg	22%
Calcium 30mg	17%
Iron 8mg	110%
Potassium 12mg	2%

Ingredients:

2 lbs or 900 g good cooking apples

4 oz or 50 g almonds (chopped)

2 oz or 50 g currants and sultanas mixed

1 stick cinnamon (about 3 inches or 7 cm long)

Juice of ½ a lemon

Whole bread (cut very thinly) spread

Sugar to taste.

Instructions:

1.	Pare, core, and cut up the apples.

2.	Stew the apples with a teacupful of water and the cinnamon, until the apples have become a pulp.

3.	Remove the cinnamon, and add sugar, lemon juice, the almonds, and the currants and sultanas (previously picked, washed, and dried).

4.	Mix all well and allow the mixture to cool.

5.	Grease a pie-dish and line it with thin slices of bread and butter,

6.	Then place on it a layer of apple mixture, repeat the layers, finishing with slices of bread and vegan butter.

7.	Bake at 375°F, 190°C or gas mark 5 for 45 minutes.

Mixed Berries Smoothie

Serving: 2

Prep Time: 4 minutes

Cook Time: 0 minutes

Ingredients:

¼ cup frozen blueberries

¼ cup frozen blackberries

1 cup unsweetened almond milk

1 teaspoon vanilla bean extract

3 teaspoons flaxseeds

1 scoop chilled Greek yogurt

Stevia as needed

How To:

1.   Mix everything in a blender and emulsify.

2.   Pulse the mixture four time until you have your desired thickness.

3.   Pour the mixture into a glass and enjoy!

Nutrition (Per Serving)

Calories: 221

Fat: 9g

Protein: 21g

Carbohydrates: 10g

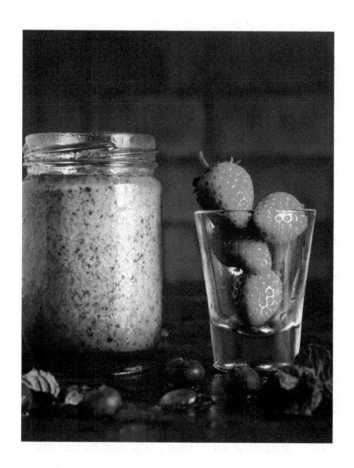

Satisfying Berry and Almond Smoothie

Serving: 4

Prep Time: 10 minutes

Cook Time: nil

Ingredients:

1 cup blueberries, frozen

1 whole banana

½ cup almond milk

1 tablespoon almond butter

Water as needed

How To:

1.   Add the listed ingredients to your blender and blend well until you have a smoothie-like texture.

2.   Chill and serve.

3.   Enjoy!

Nutrition (Per Serving)

Calories: 321

Fat: 11g

Carbohydrates: 55g

Protein: 5g

Simple Rice Mushroom Risotto

Serving: 4

Prep Time: 5 minutes

Cook Time: 15 minutes

Ingredients:

4 ½ cups cauliflower, riced

3 tablespoons coconut oil

1-pound Portobello mushrooms, thinly sliced

1-pound white mushrooms, thinly sliced

2 shallots, diced

¼ cup organic vegetable broth

Sunflower seeds and pepper to taste

3 tablespoons chives, chopped

4 tablespoons almond butter

½ cup kite ricotta/cashew cheese, grated

How To:

1.   Use a food processor and pulse cauliflower florets until riced.

2.   Take a large saucepan and heat up 2 tablespoons oil over medium-high flame.

3.   Add mushrooms and sauté for 3 minutes until mushrooms are tender.

4.   Clear saucepan of mushrooms and liquid and keep them on the side.

5.   Add the rest of the 1 tablespoon oil to skillet.

6.   Toss shallots and cook for 60 seconds.

7.   Add cauliflower rice, stir for 2 minutes until coated with oil.

8.   Add broth to riced cauliflower and stir for 5 minutes.

9.   Remove pot from heat and mix in mushrooms and liquid.

10.   Add chives, almond butter, parmesan cheese.

11.   Season with sunflower seeds and pepper.

12.   Serve and enjoy!

Nutrition (Per Serving)

Calories: 438

Fat: 17g

Carbohydrates: 15g

Protein: 12g

Hearty Green Bean Roast

Serving: 4

Prep Time: 10 minutes

Cook Time: 20 minutes

Ingredients:

1 whole egg

2 tablespoons olive oil

Sunflower seeds and pepper to taste

1-pound fresh green beans

5 ½ tablespoons grated parmesan cheese

How To:

1.   Pre-heat your oven to 400 degrees F.

2.   Take a bowl and whisk in eggs with oil and spices.

3.   Add beans and mix well.

4.   Stir in parmesan cheese and pour the mix into baking pan (lined with parchment paper).

5.   Bake for 15-20 minutes.

6.   Serve warm and enjoy!

Nutrition (Per Serving)

Calories: 216

Fat: 21g

Carbohydrates: 7g

Protein: 9g

Almond and Blistered Beans

Serving: 4

Prep Time: 10 minutes

Cook Time: 20 minutes

Ingredients:

1-pound fresh green beans, ends trimmed

1 ½ tablespoon olive oil

¼ teaspoon sunflower seeds

1 ½ tablespoons fresh dill, minced

Juice of 1 lemon

¼ cup crushed almonds

Sunflower seeds as needed

How To:

1.   Pre-heat your oven to 400 degrees F.

2.   Add the green beans with your olive oil and also the sunflower seeds.

3.   Then spread them in one single layer on a large sized sheet pan.

4.   Roast it for 10 minutes and stir, then roast for another 8-10 minutes.

5.   Remove from the oven and keep stirring in the lemon juice alongside the dill.

6.   Top it with crushed almonds and some flaked sunflower seeds and serve.

Nutrition (Per Serving)

Calories: 347

Fat: 16g

Carbohydrates: 6g

Protein: 45g

Tomato Platter

Serving: 8

Prep Time: 10 minutes + Chill time

Cook Time: Nil

Ingredients:

1/3 cup olive oil

1 teaspoon sunflower seeds

2 tablespoons onion, chopped

¼ teaspoon pepper

½ a garlic, minced

1 tablespoon fresh parsley, minced

3 large fresh tomatoes, sliced

1 teaspoon dried basil

¼ cup red wine vinegar

How To:

1.   Take a shallow dish and arrange tomatoes in the dish.

2.   Add the rest of the ingredients in a mason jar, cover the jar and shake it well.

3.   Pour the mix over tomato slices.

4.   Let it chill for 2-3 hours.

5.   Serve!

Nutrition (Per Serving)

Calories: 350

Fat: 28g

Carbohydrates: 10g

Protein: 14g

Fudge Brownies

Nutritional Facts

servings per container	9
Prep Total	**10 min**
Serving Size 2/3 cup (70g)	
Amount per serving **Calories**	**10**
	% Daily Value
Total Fat 20g	**2%**
Saturated Fat 2g	10%
Trans Fat 4g	-
Cholesterol	**10%**
Sodium 50mg	**12%**
Total Carbohydrate 7g	**20%**
Dietary Fiber 4g	7%
Total Sugar 12g	-
Protein 3g	
Vitamin C 2mcg	19%
Calcium 260mg	20%
Iron 8mg	8%
Potassium 235mg	6%

Ingredients

2 cups flour

2 cups of sugar

½ cup of cocoa powder

1 teaspoon baking powder

½ teaspoon salt

1 cup of vegetable oil

1 cup of water

1 teaspoon vanilla

1 cup dairy-free chocolate chips (optional)

½ cup chopped walnuts (optional)

Instructions:

1. Preheat oven to 350°F and grease a 9 x 13-inch baking pan.

2. Add dry ingredients in a mixing bowl. Whisk together wet ingredients and fold into the dry ingredients.

3. If desired, add half the chocolate chips and chopped walnuts to the mix. Pour mixture into the prepared pan and sprinkle with remaining chocolate chips and walnuts, if using.

4. For fudge-like brownies, bake for 20-25 minutes. For cake-like brownies, bake 25-30 minutes. Let the brownies cool slightly before serving.

Pomegranate Quinoa Porridge

Nutritional Facts

servings per container	4
Prep Total	**10 min**
Serving Size 2/3 cup (40g)	
Amount per serving **Calories**	**22**
	% Daily Value
Total Fat 12g	**20%**
Saturated Fat 2g	4%
Trans Fat 01g	1.22%
Cholesterol	**22%**
Sodium 170mg	**10%**
Total Carbohydrate 34g	**22%**
Dietary Fiber 5g	14%
Total Sugar 7g	-
Protein 3g	
Vitamin C 2mcg	10%
Calcium 260mg	20%
Iron 0mg	40%
Potassium 235mg	6%

Ingredients

1 1/2 cup quinoa flakes

2 1/2 teaspoons cinnamon

1 teaspoon vanilla extract

10 organic pDashes, pitted and cut into 1/4's

1 pomegranate pulp

1/4 cup desiccated coconut

Stewed apples

Coconut flakes to garnish

Instructions:

1.   Gently place quinoa & almond milk into saucepan, & stir on medium to low heat for 9 minutes, until it smooth

2.   Include cinnamon, desiccated coconut & vanilla extract & taste

3.   Pit pDashes & cut into quarters include to porridge stir in well

4.   Serve into individual bowls

5.   Add a scoop of stewed apple (kindly view recipe below), pomegranates, pDashes & coconut flakes

Cinnamon and Coconut Porridge

Serving: 4

Prep Time: 5 minutes

Cook Time: 5 minutes

Ingredients:

1 cup water

1/2 cup 36-percent low-fat cream

½ cup unsweetened dried coconut, shredded 1 tablespoon oat bran

1 tablespoon flaxseed meal

1/2 tablespoon almond butter

1 ½ teaspoons stevia

½ teaspoon cinnamon

Toppings, such as blueberries or banana slices

How To:

1.   Add the ingredients to alittle pot and blend well until fully incorporated

2.   Transfer the pot to your stove over medium-low heat and convey the combination to a slow boil.

3.   Stir well and take away from the warmth .

4.   Divide the mixture into equal servings and allow them to sit for 10 minutes.

5.   Top together with your desired toppings and enjoy!

Nutrition (Per Serving)

Calories: 171

Fat: 16g

Protein: 2g

Carbohydrates: 8g

Coconut Porridge

Serving: 2

Prep Time: 15 minutes

Cook Time: Nil

Ingredients:

2 tablespoons coconut flour

2 tablespoons vanilla protein powder

3 tablespoons Golden Flaxseed meal

1 ½ cups almond milk, unsweetened

Powdered Erythritol

How To:

1.   Take a bowl and blend within the flaxseed meal, protein powder, coconut flour and blend well.

2.   Add the combination to the saucepan (placed over medium heat).

3.   Add almond milk and stir, let the mixture thicken.

4.   Add your required amount of sweetener and serve.

5.   Enjoy!

Nutrition (Per Serving)

Calories: 259

Fat: 13g

Carbohydrates: 5g

Protein: 16g

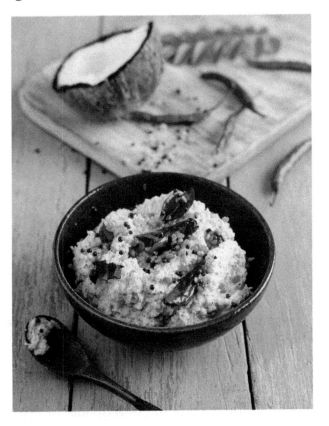

Cinnamon Pear Oatmeal

Serving: 2

Prep Time: 10 minutes

Cook Time: 15 minutes

Ingredients:

3 cups water

1 cup steel-cut oats

1 tablespoon cinnamon powder

1 cup pear, cored and peeled, cubed

How To:

1.   Take a pot and add the water, oats, cinnamon, pear and toss well.

2.   Bring it to simmer over medium heat.

3.   Let it cook for quarter-hour , and divide into two bowls.

4.   Enjoy!

Nutrition (Per Serving)

Calories: 171

Fat: 5g

Carbohydrates: 11g

Protein: 6g

Banana and Walnut Bowl

Serving: 4

Prep Time: 10 minutes

Cook Time: 15 minutes

Ingredients:

2 cups water

1 cup steel-cut oats

1 cup almond milk

¼ cup walnuts, chopped

2 tablespoons chia seeds

2 bananas, peeled and mashed

1 teaspoon vanilla flavoring

How To:

1. Take a pot and add all ingredients, toss well.

2. Bring it to simmer over medium heat.

3. Let it cook for quarter-hour , and divide into 4 bowls.

4. Enjoy!

Nutrition (Per Serving)

Calories: 162

Fat: 4g

Carbohydrates: 11g

Protein: 4g

Scrambled Pesto Eggs

Serving: 2

Prep Time: 5 minutes

Cook Time: 5 minutes

Ingredients:

2 large whole eggs

1/2 tablespoon almond butter

1/2 tablespoon pesto

1 tablespoon creamed coconut

almond milk

Sunflower seeds and pepper as needed

How To:

1.   Take a bowl and crack open your eggs.

2.   Season with a pinch of sunflower seeds and pepper.

3.   Pour eggs into a pan.

4.   Add almond butter and introduce heat.

5.   Cook on low heat and gently add pesto.

6.   Once the eggs are cooked and scrambled, remove from the warmth.

7.   Spoon in coconut milk and blend well.

8.   activate the warmth and cook on LOW for a short time until you've got a creamy texture.

9. Serve and enjoy!

Nutrition (Per Serving)

Calories: 467

Fat: 41g

Carbohydrates: 3g

Protein: 20g

Barley Porridge

Serving: 4

Prep Time: 5 minutes

Cook Time: 25 minutes

Ingredients:

1 cup barley

1 cup wheat berries

2 cups unsweetened almond milk

2 cups water

Toppings, such as hazelnuts, honey, berry, etc.

How To:

1.   Take a medium saucepan and place it over medium-high heat.

2.   Place barley, almond milk, wheat berries, water and convey to a boil.

3.   Lower the warmth to low and simmer for 25 minutes.

4.   Divide amongst serving bowls and top together with your

desired toppings.

5.   Serve and enjoy!

Nutrition (Per Serving)

Calories: 295

Fat: 8g

Carbohydrates: 56g

Protein: 6g

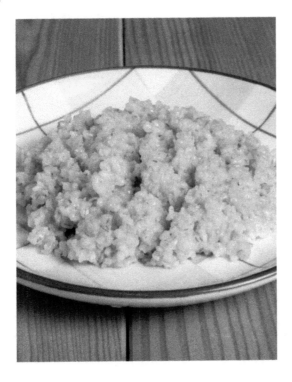

Mustard Chicken

Serving: 2

Prep Time: 10 minutes

Cook Time: 40 minutes

Ingredients:

2 chicken breasts

1/4 cup chicken broth

2 tablespoons mustard

1 1/2 tablespoons olive oil

1/2 teaspoon paprika

1/2 teaspoon chili powder

1/2 teaspoon garlic powder

How To:

1.   Take alittle bowl and blend mustard, olive oil, paprika, chicken stock, garlic powder, chicken stock , and chili.

2.   Add pigeon breast and marinate for half-hour .

3.   Take a lined baking sheet and arrange the chicken.

4.   Bake for 35 minutes at 375 degrees F.

5.   Serve and enjoy!

Nutrition (Per Serving)

Calories: 531

Fat: 23g

Carbohydrates: 10g

Protein: 64g

Chicken and Carrot Stew

Serving: 4

Prep Time: 15 minutes

Cook Time: 6 hours

Ingredients:

4 boneless chicken breast, cubed

3 cups of carrots, peeled and cubed

1 cup onion, chopped

1 cup tomatoes, chopped

1 teaspoon of dried thyme

2 cups of chicken broth

2 garlic cloves, minced

Sunflower seeds and pepper as needed

How To:

1.   Add all of the listed ingredients to a Slow Cooker.

2.   Stir and shut the lid.

3.   Cook for six hours.

4.   Serve hot and enjoy!

Nutrition (Per Serving)

Calories: 182

Fat: 3g

Carbohydrates: 10g

Protein: 39g

The Delish Turkey Wrap

Serving: 6

Prep Time: 10 minutes

Cook Time: 10 minutes

Ingredients:

1 ¼ pounds ground turkey, lean

4 green onions, minced

1 tablespoon olive oil

1 garlic clove, minced

2 teaspoons chili paste

8-ounce water chestnut, diced

3 tablespoons hoisin sauce

2 tablespoon coconut aminos

1 tablespoon rice vinegar

12 almond butter lettuce leaves

1/8 teaspoon sunflower seeds

How To:

1.   Take a pan and place it over medium heat, add turkey and garlic to the pan.

2.   Heat for six minutes until cooked.

3.   Take a bowl and transfer turkey to the bowl.

4.   Add onions and water chestnuts.

5.   Stir in duck sauce , coconut aminos, vinegar and chili paste.

6.   Toss well and transfer mix to lettuce leaves.

7.   Serve and enjoy!

Nutrition (Per Serving)

Calories: 162

Fat: 4g

Net Carbohydrates: 7g

Protein: 23g

Almond Butternut Chicken

Serving: 4

Prep Time: 15 minutes

Cook Time: 30 minutes

Ingredients:

½ pound Nitrate free bacon

6 chicken thighs, boneless and skinless

2-3 cups almond butternut squash, cubed Extra virgin olive oil
Fresh chopped sage

Sunflower seeds and pepper as needed

How To:

1.   Prepare your oven by preheating it to 425 degrees F.

2.   Take an outsized skillet and place it over medium-high
heat, add bacon and fry until crispy.

3.   Take a slice of bacon and place it on the side, crumble the
bacon.

4.   Add cubed almond butternut squash within the bacon
grease and sauté, season with sunflower seeds and pepper.

5.   Once the squash is tender, remove skillet and transfer to a plate.

6.   Add copra oil to the skillet and add chicken thighs, cook for 10 minutes.

7.   Season with sunflower seeds and pepper.

8.   Remove skillet from stove and transfer to oven.

9.   Bake for 12-15 minutes, top with the crumbled bacon and sage.

10.   Enjoy!

Nutrition (Per Serving)

Calories: 323

Fat: 19g

Carbohydrates: 8g

Protein: 12g

Zucchini Zoodles with Chicken and Basil

Serving: 3

Prep Time: 10 minutes

Cook Time: 10 minutes

Ingredients:

2 chicken fillets, cubed

2 tablespoons ghee

1-pound tomatoes, diced

½ cup basil, chopped

¼ cup almond milk

1 garlic clove, peeled, minced

1 zucchini, shredded

How To:

1. Sauté cubed chicken in ghee until not pink.

2. Add tomatoes and season with sunflower seeds.

3. Simmer and reduce liquid.

4. Prepare your zucchini Zoodles by shredding zucchini during a kitchen appliance .

5. Add basil, garlic, coconut almond milk to the chicken and cook for a couple of minutes.

6. Add half the zucchini Zoodles to a bowl and top with creamy tomato basil chicken.

7. Enjoy!

Nutrition (Per Serving)

Calories: 540

Fat: 27g

Carbohydrates: 13g

Protein: 59g

Beef Soup

Serving: 4

Prep Time: 10 minutes

Cook Time: 40 minutes

Ingredients:

1-pound ground beef, lean

1 cup mixed vegetables, frozen

1 yellow onion, chopped

6 cups vegetable broth

1 cup low-fat cream Pepper to taste

How To:

1.   Take a stockpot and add all the ingredients the except cream, salt, and black pepper.

2.   bring back a boil.

3.   Reduce heat to simmer.

4.   Cook for 40 minutes.

5.   Once cooked, warm the cream .

6. Then add once the soup is cooked.

7. Blend the soup till smooth by using an immersion blender.

8. Season with salt and black pepper.

9. Serve and enjoy!

Nutrition (Per Serving)

Calories: 270

Fat: 14g

Carbohydrates: 6g

Protein: 29g

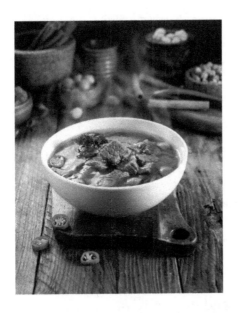

Amazing Grilled Chicken and Blueberry Salad

Serving: 5

Prep Time: 10 minutes

Cook Time: 25 minutes

Smart Points: 9

Ingredients:

5 cups mixed greens

1 cup blueberries

¼ cup slivered almonds

2 cups chicken breasts, cooked and cubed

For dressing

¼ cup olive oil

¼ cup apple cider vinegar

¼ cup blueberries

2 tablespoons honey

Sunflower seeds and pepper to taste

How To:

1.   Take a bowl and add greens, berries, almonds, chicken cubes and blend well.

2.   Take a bowl and blend the dressing ingredients, pour the combination into a blender and blitz until smooth.

3.   Add dressing on top of the chicken cubes and toss well.

4.   Season more and enjoy!

Nutrition (Per Serving)

Calories: 266

Fat: 17g

Carbohydrates: 18g

Protein: 10g

Clean Chicken and Mushroom Stew

Serving: 4

Prep Time: 10 minutes

Cook Time: 35 minutes

Ingredients:

4 chicken breast halves, cut into bite sized pieces

1 pound mushrooms, sliced (5-6 cups)

1 bunch spring onion, chopped

4 tablespoons olive oil

1 teaspoon thyme

Sunflower seeds and pepper as needed

How To:

1.   Take an outsized deep frypan and place it over medium-high heat.

2.   Add oil and let it heat up.

3.   Add chicken and cook for 4-5 minutes per side until slightly browned.

4.   Add spring onions and mushrooms, season with sunflower seeds and pepper consistent with your taste.

5.   Stir.

6.   Cover with lid and convey the combination to a boil.

7.   Reduce heat and simmer for 25 minutes.

8.   Serve!

Nutrition (Per Serving)

Calories: 247

Fat: 12g

Carbohydrates: 10g

Protein: 23g

Elegant Pumpkin Chili Dish

Serving: 4

Prep Time: 10 minutes

Cook Time: 15 minutes

Ingredients:

3 cups yellow onion, chopped

8 garlic cloves, chopped

1 pound turkey, ground

2 cans (15 ounces each) fire roasted tomatoes

2 cups pumpkin puree

1 cup chicken broth

4 teaspoons chili spice

1 teaspoon ground cinnamon

1 teaspoon sea sunflower seeds

How To:

1.   Take an outsized sized pot and place it over medium-high heat.

2.   Add copra oil and let the oil heat up.

3.   Add onion and garlic, sauté for five minutes.

4.   Add ground turkey and break it while cooking, cook for five minutes.

5.   Add remaining ingredients and convey the combination to simmer.

6.   Simmer for quarter-hour over low heat (lid off).

7.   Pour chicken stock .

8.   Serve with desired salad.

9.   Enjoy!

Nutrition (Per Serving)

Calories: 312

Fat: 16g

Carbohydrates: 14g

Protein: 27g

Simple Garlic and Lemon Soup

Serving: 3

Prep Time: 10 minutes

Cook Time: nil

Ingredients:

1 avocado, pitted and chopped

1 cucumber, chopped

2 bunches spinach

1 ½ cups watermelon, chopped

1 bunch cilantro, roughly chopped

Juice from 2 lemons

½ cup coconut amines

½ cup lime juice

How To:

1.   Add cucumber, avocado to your blender and pulse well.

2.   Add cilantro, spinach and watermelon and blend.

3.   Add lemon, juice and coconut amino.

4.   Pulse a couple of more times.

5.   Transfer to bowl and enjoy!

Nutrition (Per Serving)

Calories: 100

Fat: 7g

Carbohydrates: 6g

Protein: 3g

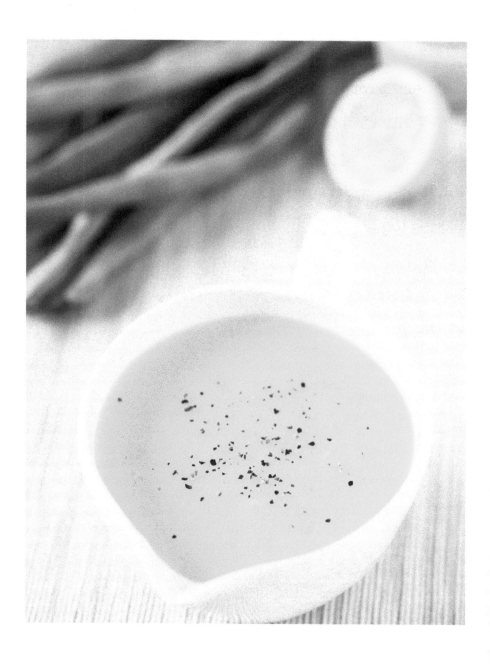

Healthy Cucumber Soup

Serving: 4

Prep Time: 14 minutes

Cook Time: Nil

Ingredients:

2 tablespoons garlic, minced

4 cups English cucumbers, peeled and diced ½ cup onions, diced

1 tablespoon lemon juice 1 ½ cups vegetable broth ½ teaspoon sunflower seeds ¼ teaspoon red pepper flakes

¼ cup parsley, diced

½ cup Greek yogurt, plain

How To:

1.   Add the listed ingredients to a blender and blend to emulsify (keep aside ½ cup of chopped cucumbers).

2.   Blend until smooth.

3.   Divide the soup amongst 4 servings and top with extra cucumbers.

4.   Enjoy chilled!

Nutrition (Per Serving)

Calories: 371

Fat: 36g

Carbohydrates: 8g

Protein: 4g

Mushroom Cream Soup

Serving: 4

Prep Time: 5 minutes

Cook Time: 30 minutes

Ingredients:

1 tablespoon olive oil

½ large onion, diced

20 ounces mushrooms, sliced

6 garlic cloves, minced

2 cups vegetable broth

1 cup coconut cream

¾ teaspoon sunflower seeds

¼ teaspoon black pepper

1 cup almond milk

How To:

1. Take an outsized sized pot and place it over medium heat.

2.   Add onion and mushrooms to the vegetable oil and sauté for 10-15 minutes.

3.   confirm to stay stirring it from time to time until browned evenly.

4.   Add garlic and sauté for 10 minutes more.

5.   Add vegetable broth, coconut milk , almond milk[MOU6], black pepper and sunflower seeds.

6.   Bring it to a boil and lower the temperature to low.

7.   Simmer for quarter-hour .

8.   Use an immersion blender to puree the mixture.

9.   Enjoy!

Nutrition (Per Serving)

Calories: 200

Fat: 17g

Carbohydrates: 5g

Protein: 4g

Curious Roasted Garlic Soup

Serving: 10

Prep Time: 10 minutes

Cook Time: 60 minutes

Ingredients:

1 tablespoon olive oil

2 bulbs garlic, peeled

3 shallots, chopped

1 large head cauliflower, chopped

6 cups vegetable broth

Sunflower seeds and pepper to taste

How To:

1.   Pre-heat your oven to 400 degrees F.

2.   Slice ¼ inch top of garlic bulb and place it in aluminum foil.

3.   Grease with vegetable oil and roast in oven for 35 minutes.

4. Squeeze flesh out of the roasted garlic.

5. Heat oil in saucepan and add shallots, sauté for six minutes.

6. Add garlic and remaining ingredients.

7. Cover pan and reduce heat to low.

8. Let it cook for 15-20 minutes.

9. Use an immersion blender to puree the mixture. 10. Season soup with sunflower seeds and pepper.

10. Serve and enjoy!

Nutrition (Per Serving)

Calories: 142

Fat: 8g

Carbohydrates: 3.4g

Protein: 4g

Amazing Roasted Carrot Soup

Serving: 4

Prep Time: 10 minutes

Cook Time: 50 minutes

Ingredients:

8 large carrots, washed and peeled

6 tablespoons olive oil

1-quart broth

Cayenne pepper to taste

Sunflower seeds and pepper to taste

How To:

1.   Pre-heat your oven to 425 degrees F.

2.   Take a baking sheet and add carrots, drizzle vegetable oil and roast for 30-45 minutes.

3.   Put roasted carrots into blender and add broth, puree.

4.   Pour into saucepan and warmth soup.

5.   Season with sunflower seeds, pepper and cayenne.

6.   Drizzle vegetable oil .

7.   Serve and enjoy!

Nutrition (Per Serving)

Calories: 222

Fat: 18g

Net Carbohydrates: 7g

Protein: 5g

Simple Pumpkin Soup

Serving: 4

Prep Time: 5 minutes

Cook Time: 6-8 hours

Ingredients:

1 small pumpkin, halved, peeled, seeds removed, cubed

2 cups chicken broth

1 cup coconut milk

Pepper and thyme to taste

How To:

1. Add all the ingredients to a crockpot.

2. Close the lid.

3. Cook for 6-8 hours on low.

4. Make a smooth puree by employing a blender.

5. Garnish with roasted seeds.

6. Serve and enjoy!

Nutrition (Per Serving)

Calories: 60

Fat: 2g

Net Carbohydrates: 10g

Protein: 3g

Coconut Avocado Soup

Serving: 4

Prep Time: 5 minutes

Cook Time: 5-10 minutes

Ingredients:

2 cups vegetable stock

2 teaspoons Thai green curry paste

Pepper as needed

1 avocado, chopped

1 tablespoon cilantro, chopped

Lime wedges

1 cup coconut milk

How To:

1.   Add milk, avocado, curry paste, pepper to blender and blend.

2.   Take a pan and place it over medium heat.

3.   Add mixture and warmth , simmer for five minutes.

4.   Stir in seasoning, cilantro and simmer for 1 minute.

5.   Serve and enjoy!

Nutrition (Per Serving)

Calories: 250

Fat: 30g

Net Carbohydrates: 2g

Protein: 4g

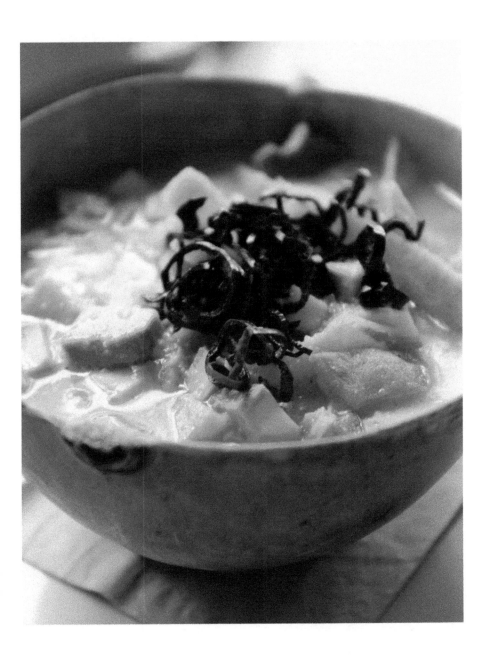

Lightning Source UK Ltd.
Milton Keynes UK
UKHW020652240521
384262UK00001B/64